THREE WEEK
STEP INTO A
HEALTHIER YOU

Lourdes Lavoy

I dedicate this to all those who have reached out to me and asked if I could write a book on things they could do daily to improve their health and food intake.

CONTENTS

NOTES

_____
_____
_____
_____
_____
_____
_____
_____
_____
_____
_____
_____
_____
_____
_____
_____
_____
_____
_____
_____
_____
_____
_____

THREE WEEK STEP INTO A HEALTHIER YOU
by
Lourdes Lavoy

Dedicated to your health

We live in a world that keeps us on the busiest of schedules. We must find a less complex way to give our bodies a thriving chance at a healthier life. With that goal in mind, I decided to put this book together. The idea came as sort of an inspiration: Create a book that will give you a three-week schedule to manifest healthier habits with your diet. The book is designed to give daily, practical guidance. The plan is simplified by design so that baby steps can be taken to a new you.

At the beginning of each week, I will provide a list of ingredients. I will also explain why the ingredient is on the list and its health benefits. There will be some repetition in ingredients, and you will see benefits listed from the prior week; the goal is to get you familiar with the health benefits.

The goal here is to first build a foundation and then to add a new ingredient daily adding onto the foundation. When I was faced with the necessity to adhere to a strict diet to fight my Hodgkin's Lymphoma the experience was overwhelming. Suddenly there was a monumental list of new foods to get my health back on track. My goal then is to slowly introduce more ingredients to the already established list of ingredients in an attempt to not overwhelm anyone looking to improve their health. It's like slowly easing into a hot tub, as to not scald in one dunk. On the sixth day of each week, lunch will be added to the list. On the seventh day of each week, lunch, and dinner will both be added to the list. Cheers to your health.

INGREDIENTS FOR THE FIRST WEEK

So as to not overwhelm anyone and get into a good healthy habit; we will start each day with one new ingredient added to your daily intake. Note that many of the ingredients will have much more compounds that do so much more than I can put in one page. But I'm here to give you the general idea of how good these foods are for your overall health; one is that all of the ingredients in this book help keep your blood sugar levels low in their normal way.

BENEFITS

Lemons contain high levels of vitamin C and are quite effective in curing digestion problems. They also carry digestive juices that relieve you from things like heartburn, bloating, belching, and gastric problems. By taking lemon with fresh warm water in the morning, it aids in proper digestion. It removes toxins from the kidneys and the digestive system. It is good for high blood pressure, Cold and fevers, respiratory disorders, dental health, weight loss, and so much more.

Celery is great in hydration; it also contains vitamins A, K, C, E, and B vitamins. It carries compounds that may help with inflammation in the body, help in lowering cholesterol levels and reduce blood pressure. Boost the immune system and reduce pain. The list is way too long, but you get the picture.

Green apples promote weight loss, improves hair quality, great for skin health, protect our vision, and improve digestion. Digestion is key to our overall health, as it is through our digestion that we receive our nutrition. If we have joint problems, green apples have been known to strengthen our joints. Green apples are also known to detoxify the liver. This is important since the liver does over five hundred functions for the body. Now we can see why the old saying goes *An Apple a Day Keeps the Doctor Away.* I mean, when you look up information on the health benefits of green apples, we also learn it can prevent asthma, strengthens the immune system, and on and on it goes.

Kale contains Vitamins A, K, C, B6, Manganese, Calcium, Copper, Potassium, and Magnesium, to name a few. Magnesium alone is amazing because its mineral helps the cells communicate with each other, so they all do their jobs. High in antioxidants is a plus. It is an excellent source of vitamin C. It is also great for the heart and so much more.

Cucumbers are packed with a lot of important nutrients our bodies require to function well.

Cucumber carries vitamin C, K, Magnesium, Potassium (that many seem to be low on), and Manganese. They also contain antioxidants and micronutrients. And again great for blood pressure and keeps the digestion going strong.

Berries (Raspberries, blackberries, strawberries, and blueberries) are loaded with antioxidants, keeping free radicals under control. They help improve blood sugar and insulin response. They are high in fiber. They are high in vitamin C, Manganese, vitamin K1, Copper, and Folate. They fight inflammation, may help lower cholesterol levels, and are great for the skin. And because of their high antioxidants, they may help protect against cancer.

Avocado is incredibly nutritious. Some of the nutrients; vitamin K, Folate, vitamin C, Potassium, vitamin B5, vitamin B6, and vitamin E, to name a few. Avocados are loaded with fiber. Eating avocados can lower your cholesterol and triglyceride levels and may even relieve symptoms of arthritis.

Leafy greens support brain function, make your skin glow, relieve stress, support bone health, boost digestive enzymes, and support the immune system. You can find many studies on the health benefits of eating leafy greens. You have a variety to pick from. I personally love mixing several. Here are a few to list, kale, spinach, arugula, and chard, to name a few.

Seeds, such as flax seeds, chia seeds, pumpkin, and sunflower, carry omegas along with fiber, protein and magnesium. That is just a few of many things they carry. Seeds are a great source of healthy fats and proteins along with antioxidants to help keep you healthy.

Cucumber, carry protein, fiber, vitamin C, vitamin K, magnesium, and potassium. Cucumbers also contain antioxidants that block oxidation. It promotes hydration and may aid in weight loss and lower blood sugar.

Purple rice, also known as black rice, can be purchased by just typing in purple rice on the internet. My favorite is called Forbidden black rice. It is sold in many stores in the rice section. Black rice is high in protein and is also a good source of iron. It is rich in antioxidants, anti-inflammatory, and has anti-cancer effects. May boost and support heart health and eye health. It is gluten-free for those who are watching their gluten intake. And yes, it is known to lower blood sugar levels.

Eggplant is rich in many nutrients. It has fiber, protein, potassium, folate, vitamin K, and vitamin C. They are high in antioxidants and may reduce the risk of heart disease.

Broccoli, packed with vitamins, minerals, and bioactive compounds are known to prevent cellular damage in the eyes, reduce blood sugar, cholesterol levels, and reduce inflammation. And the biggie protects against certain cancers.

Onions that is high in vitamin C is involved in regulating immune health, collagen production, tissue repair, and the absorption of iron.

Melons carry anti-cancer compounds; they can stop the clotting of blood cells that cause strokes or heart disease. They are beneficial in healing kidney disease and amazing for your digestive health. It also has anti-aging benefits and promotes hair growth.

Quinoa is a very nutritious grain. There are three main types: white, red, and black. It is high in protein. Has fiber, Manganese, Magnesium, Phosphorus, Folate, Copper, Iron, Zinc, Potassium, and over 10% of the RDA for vitamins B1, B2, and B6.

Sea salt, not all salt is created equal, and there is a difference between unrefined, mineral-rich varieties like sea salt versus salt that has been heavily processed and stripped of its natural nutrients. Sea salts are a great source of micronutrients. Sea salt contains many of the major electrolytes, like sodium, magnesium, calcium, and potassium, essential to good health. Regular table salt is stripped from those essential nutrients.

Grapes have been associated with the prevention of cancer, heart disease, high blood pressure, and constipation. The nutrients in grapes may help protect against cancer, eye problems, and cardiovascular disease. Grapes are also known to help with fatigue, kidney disorders, macular degeneration, and the prevention of cataracts.

Mixed vegetables are going to be used for your lunch. Pick your favorite mixed veggies.

Behold, I have given you every plant yielding seed that is on the surface of all the earth, and every tree which has fruit yielding seed; it shall be food for you.

Genesis 1:29

WEEK ONE - DAY ONE

Each day may seem repetitive, but it is in the repetition that we create habits. This book is all about healthy habits. Now let's get started.

No matter where you are in your life when it comes to health you can always benefit from good nutritional habits.

We will start each day with an affirmation. For the next 21 days, we will go on a ride together of new beginnings. For some, this won't be as new to you, but rather it becomes a bonus to what you already do.

Every morning for the next 21 days, when you wake up, really feel the gratitude for the health you have at this moment. Remember, you are alive and above ground. That is always a good day.

Step one starts your affirmation by looking in the mirror and saying <u>thank you for my healthy body,</u> then ends it with <u>thank you, thank you, thank you.</u> I really feel it when you say it.

Next, after you have done your morning hygiene, squeeze a half lemon into a glass of drinking water, about 4 ounces or more. Store the other half in a container and refrigerate it for tomorrow. *Wait about 10 minutes before drinking or eating anything else.* For <u>breakfast,</u> make a bowl of berries and mix with some vegan yogurt made from coconut. Read ahead, so you know what you will need for day two.

Do three simple exercises, then write down the number of reps you did for each one on the next page.

NOTES

Non-violence leads to the highest ethics, which is the goal of all evolution. Until we stop harming all other living beings, we are still savages...

Thomas A. Edison

WEEK ONE - DAY TWO

Step one: start your affirmation, look in the mirror and say <u>thank you for my healthy body,</u> then end it with <u>thank you, thank you, thank you.</u>

Next, after you have done your morning hygiene, squeeze a half lemon into a glass of drinking water, about 4 ounces or more. *Wait about 10 minutes before drinking the fresh celery juice you are about to make for <u>breakfast</u>.*

In your juicer, preferably a masticating juicer, juice 4 stems of celery. *After drinking your juice, wait at least an hour before eating anything else;* a bowl of fruit would be ideal. Each day we will be adding a new ingredient to the juice, so make sure you have got all the ingredients listed above or read ahead, so you know what you will need for the next day. For snacks, have a cup of grapes.

Do three simple exercises, then write down the number of reps you did for each one on the next page.

NOTES

All beings tremble before violence. All fear death. All love life. See yourself in others. Then whom can you hurt? What harm can you do?...

Gautama Buddha

WEEK ONE - DAY THREE

Step one: start your affirmation, look in the mirror and say thank you for my healthy body, then end it with thank you, thank you, thank you.

Next, after you have done your morning hygiene; squeeze a half lemon into a glass of drinking water, about 4 ounces or more. Use the other half of the lemon for your juice. *Wait about 10 minutes before drinking the fresh celery, lemon, and apple juice you are about to make for breakfast.*

In your juicer, juice 4 stems of celery, half of the lemon, and 1 green apple. After drinking your juice again, wait at least an hour before eating anything else. For snacks, have a cup of berries. Read ahead, so you know what you will need for tomorrow. As the week goes on, we will be adding to your juice and lunch and eventually dinner. I hope that in taking it slowly, you will have gotten into the habit of each step, hopefully making it second nature.

Do three simple exercises, then write down the number of reps you did for each one on the next page.

NOTES

_____
_____
_____
_____
_____
_____
_____
_____
_____
_____
_____
_____
_____
_____
_____
_____
_____
_____
_____
_____
_____
_____
_____
_____
_____

If slaughterhouses had glass walls, everyone would be vegetarian...

Paul McCartney

WEEK ONE - DAY FOUR

Step one: start your affirmation, look in the mirror and say <u>thank you for my healthy body,</u> then end it with <u>thank you, thank you, thank you.</u>

Next, after you have done your morning hygiene; squeeze a half lemon into a glass of drinking water, about 4 ounces or more. *Wait about 10 minutes before drinking the fresh juice you are about to make for <u>breakfast</u>.*

In your juicer, juice 2 stems of celery, half a lemon, 1 green apple, and 1 kale leaf. After drinking your juice again, wait at least an hour before eating anything else. For snacks, have a cup of berries or grapes. Read ahead, so you know what you will need for tomorrow.

Do three simple exercises, then write down the number of reps you did for each one on the next page.

NOTES

Vegetarian food leaves a deep impression on our nature. If the whole world adopts vegetarianism, it can change the destiny of humankind...

Albert Einstein

WEEK ONE - DAY FIVE

Step one: start your affirmation, look in the mirror and say <u>thank you for my healthy body,</u> then end it with <u>thank you, thank you, thank you.</u>

Next, after you have done your morning hygiene, squeeze a half lemon into a glass of drinking water, about 4 ounces or more. *Wait about 10 minutes before drinking the fresh juice you are about to make for <u>breakfast.</u>*

In your juicer, juice 2 stems of celery, half a lemon, 1 green apple, 1 kale leaf, and half a cucumber. Store the other half of the cucumber in a container and refrigerate for tomorrow. After drinking your juice again, wait at least an hour before eating anything else. For snacks, have a cup of berries. Read ahead, so you know what you will need for tomorrow.

Do three simple exercises, then write down the number of reps you did for each one on the next page.

NOTES

The greatness of a nation and its moral progress can be judged by the way its animals are treated...

Mahatma Gandhi

WEEK ONE - DAY SIX

Step one: start your affirmation, look in the mirror and say <u>thank you for my healthy body,</u> then end it with <u>thank you, thank you, thank you.</u>

Next, after you have done your morning hygiene, squeeze a half lemon into a glass of drinking water, about 4 ounces or more. *Wait about 10 minutes before drinking the fresh juice you are about to make for <u>breakfast.</u>*

In your juicer, juice 2 stems of celery, half a lemon, 1 green apple, 1 kale leaf, and a half of cucumber. *After drinking your juice again, wait at least an hour before eating anything else.* For snacks, have a cup of grapes.

Side notes; if you are at work during lunchtime, then prepare your lunch the night before.

For <u>lunch,</u> take a bag of mixed vegetables and cook on the stovetop with a little bit of water for about 5 to 10 minutes and your favorite seasoning, then add to your delicious salad. Put together different leafy greens, half an avocado sliced into cubes, 2 tablespoons of your preferred seeds (pumpkin, flaxseeds, chia seeds, or sunflower) a half of cucumbers thinly sliced, and add about ¼ cup of your favorite oil, ½ a teaspoon of sea salt to taste, mine is extra virgin olive oil with Himalayan salt. You can get creative with your salads. Add tomatoes or some raisins.

About an hour after eating, have either a glass of water or a cup of your favorite tea, sweetened with raw honey. For dessert, have some melon or berries. If you choose watermelon as your melon of choice, don't get rid of the seed. Eat them together with your watermelon, they have a nutty taste, and it's good for you. It carries the mineral Magnesium, an essential nutrient needed for good health. Read ahead, so you know what you will need for tomorrow.

Do three simple exercises, then write down the number of reps you did for each one on the next page.

NOTES

_____
_____
_____
_____
_____
_____
_____
_____
_____
_____
_____
_____
_____
_____
_____
_____
_____
_____
_____
_____
_____
_____
_____

When people ask me why I don't eat meat or any other animal products, I say, 'Because they are unhealthy and they are the product of a violent and inhumane industry...

Cassey Afleck

WEEK ONE - DAY SEVEN

Step one: start your affirmation, look in the mirror and say <u>thank you for my healthy body,</u> then end it with <u>thank you, thank you, thank you.</u>

Next, after you have done your morning hygiene, squeeze a half lemon into a glass of drinking water, about 4 ounces or more. *Wait about 10 minutes before drinking the juice you are about to make for <u>breakfast</u>.*

In your juicer, juice 2 stems of celery, half a lemon, 1 green apple, 1 kale leaf, and a half of cucumber. *After drinking your juice again, wait at least an hour before eating anything else.* For snacks, have a cup of berries.

For <u>lunch,</u> prepare some quinoa. Follow the direction in the back of the package. Quinoa takes about 10 to 15 minutes to cook. Add a few tablespoons of your cooked quinoa to your delicious salad. Put together some leafy greens, half an avocado sliced into cubes, seeds (pumpkin, flaxseeds, chia seeds, or sunflower), cucumbers, and add your favorite oil with sea salt to taste. You can get creative with your salads. Add tomatoes or some raisins, or even some types of nuts.

About an hour after eating, have either a glass of water or a cup of your favorite tea, sweetened with raw honey. For dessert, have some melon or berries.

For <u>dinner,</u> we have purple rice, which is high in antioxidants and many other valuable nutrients that I have shared at the beginning of each week. To make the rice, follow instructions on the back of your rice, usually a teaspoon of sea salt for every cup of rice, and 1 ½ cups of water for every cup of rice with a little bit of organic butter. I use vegan butter, but you can use regular butter if that is what you use. Try to stick to organic.

Make a salad on the side again using olive oil and salt to taste. Cook one eggplant sautéed in organic butter or oil with one onion and season to taste. Steam broccoli for about three minutes, keeping them slightly crunchy not to overcook and lose the nutrients. About an hour after eating, have either a glass of water or a cup of your favorite tea, sweetened with raw honey.

Congratulations, you have now finished your first week, on to the next.

Read ahead, so you know what you will need for tomorrow.

Do three simple exercises, then write down the number of reps you did for each one on the next page.

NOTES

INGREDIENTS FOR THE SECOND WEEK

BENEFITS

Basil contains a good amount of minerals like Potassium, Manganese, Magnesium, and copper. It is recommended for heart health due to its high levels of beta-carotene.

Ginger boosts your immune system, relieves nausea, and has a healing effect on your digestive system. In addition, ginger reduces blood pressure and Cholesterol and stimulates the heart. Ginger is more powerful than onions or garlic. It's known to fight inflammation and viruses and destroys the cancer stem cell. It is also known to lower cholesterol.

Spinach has protein, fiber, vitamin K, C, A, Folate, a vitamin B that helps form red blood cells and DNA. It also carries Iron and magnesium. This amazing plant supports bone health and is high in antioxidants.

Celery is great in hydration; it also contains vitamins A, K, C, E, and B vitamins. It carries compounds that may help with inflammation in the body, help in lowering cholesterol levels and reduce blood pressure. Boost the immune system and reduce pain. The list is way too long, but you get the picture.

Green Apple promotes weight loss, improves hair quality, great for skin health, protects our vision, and improves digestion. Digestion is key to our overall health, as it is through our digestion that we receive our nutrition. If we have joint problems, green apples have been known to strengthen our joints. Green apples are also known to detoxify the liver. This is important since the liver does over five hundred functions for the body. Now we can see why the old saying goes *An Apple a Day Keeps the Doctor Away.* I mean, when you look up information on the health benefits of green apples, we also learn it can prevent asthma, strengthens the immune system, and on and on it goes.

Lemon contains high levels of vitamin C and is quite effective in curing digestion problems. They also carry digestive juices that relieve you from things like heartburn, bloating, belching, and gastric problems. By taking lemon with fresh warm water in the morning, it aids in proper digestion. It removes toxins from the kidneys and the digestive system. It is good for high blood pressure, Cold and fevers, respiratory disorders, dental health, weight loss, and so much more.

Beets are high in many valuable vitamins and minerals. They actually contain a bit of almost all the vitamins and minerals you need. It helps with blood pressure, athletic performance, increases oxygen, fights inflammation, supports brain health, and has anti-cancer properties.

Carrots are great for the eyes. It promotes glowing skin, boosts your immune system, improves digestion, controls blood sugar levels, prevents cancer, and cleanses the body.

Avocado is incredibly nutritious. Some of the nutrients; vitamin K, Folate, vitamin C, Potassium, vitamin B5, vitamin B6, and vitamin E, to name a few. Avocados are loaded with fiber. Eating avocados can lower your cholesterol and triglyceride levels and may even relieve symptoms of arthritis.

Leafy greens support brain function, make your skin glow, relieve stress, support bone health, boost digestive enzymes, and support the immune system. You can find many studies on the health benefits of eating leafy greens. You have a variety to pick from; I, personally, love mixing several types of leafy greens. Here are a few to list, kale, spinach, arugula, and chard, to name a few.

Tomatoes can provide about 40% of the daily recommended minimum of vitamin C. Tomatoes supply vitamin A, which supports immunity, vision, and skin health; vitamin K, which is good for your bones; and potassium, a key nutrient for heart function, muscle contractions, and maintaining healthy blood pressure and fluid balance. It's at its highest concentration when tomatoes have been cooked. You will also need a small can of **tomato paste**.

Cucumber, carry protein, fiber, vitamin C, vitamin K, magnesium, and potassium. Cucumbers also contain antioxidants that block oxidation. It promotes hydration and may aid in weight loss and lower blood sugar.

Spaghetti squash is great for the eyes, relieving high blood pressure, gout, arthritis, heart diseases, and helping in the proper functioning of the brain. It carries antioxidants, vitamin C, Anthocyanin, and Folate, as well as Quercetin. Aids in digestion and are beneficial for our skin and eyes.

Olive oil helps clear the blood of toxins, balances your cholesterol. It's anti-inflammatory, antibacterial, heart-healthy, and skin-healthy.

Garlic salt can reduce cholesterol levels, blood pressure and boost the immune system. Regular garlic supplementation can prove effective in fighting off mild infections, like the common cold. It is known as nature's antibiotic.

Quinoa is a very nutritious grain. There are three main types: white, red, and black. It is high in protein. Has fiber, Manganese, Magnesium, Phosphorus, Folate, Copper, Iron, Zinc, Potassium, and over 10% of the RDA for vitamins B1, B2, and B6.

Sea salt, not all salt is created equal, and there is a difference between unrefined, mineral-rich varieties like sea salt versus salt that has been heavily processed and stripped of their natural nutrients. Sea salts are a great source of micronutrients. Sea salt contains many of the major electrolytes, like sodium, magnesium, calcium, and potassium, essential to good health. Regular table salt is stripped from those essential nutrients.

Berries (Raspberries, blackberries, strawberries, and blueberries) are loaded with antioxidants, keeping free radicals under control. They help improve blood sugar and insulin response. They are high in fiber. They are high in vitamin C, Manganese, vitamin K1, Copper, and Folate. They fight inflammation, may help lower cholesterol levels, and are great for the skin. And because of their high antioxidants, they may help protect against cancer.

Grapes have been associated with preventing cancer, heart disease, high blood pressure, and constipation. In addition, the nutrients in grapes may help protect against cancer, eye problems, and cardiovascular disease. Grapes are also known to help with fatigue, kidney disorders, macular degeneration, and the prevention of cataracts.

Watermelon's health benefits are vast and include preventing diseases and disorders, including kidney disorders, high blood pressure, cancer, diabetes, heart diseases, heat stroke, macular degeneration, and even impotence. The watermelon seeds that you would chew up and eat are low in calories and high in nutrients, and no, they are not poisonous though they may be hard to digest for some. Instead, they boost heart health and immunity and keep your blood sugar levels under control. In addition, the seeds are rich in numerous micronutrients like potassium, copper, selenium, and zinc – nutrients that you may not obtain from your diet in adequate quantities.

Eating the seeds directly from the fruit is good, but the sprouted ones are better. Just about 1/8 cup of the seeds offers about 10 grams of protein. Sprouting the seeds also removes the compounds in the seeds that make them harder to be absorbed by the body. So if you prefer to sprout them, instead go for it but don't throw them away. I eat them fresh from the melon but sprouting them is also very beneficial.

Cabbage reduces the risk of cancer, improving brain and nervous system health, promoting bone health, maintaining blood pressure, detoxifying the body, promoting bowel regularity, regulating sugar level, and promoting weight loss. Other benefits; improves healthy hair, skin, and nails.

Zucchini contains zero fat and is high in water and fiber. It also contains significant amounts of vitamins B6, riboflavin, folate, C, and K, and minerals, like potassium and manganese. This summer squash also contains antioxidant and anti-inflammatory phytonutrients. It slows down aging and improves eye health.

Onions are high in vitamin C that is involved in regulating immune health, collagen production, tissue repair, and iron absorption.

It's the 21st century. It's healthier for us, better for the environment and certainly kinder to be a vegetarian...

Ingrid Newkirk

WEEK TWO – DAY ONE

We will always start our day with a daily affirmation and our glass of water with fresh-squeezed lemon. Let's get started.

Step one: start your affirmation, look in the mirror and say <u>thank you for my healthy body,</u> then end it with <u>thank you, thank you, thank you</u>, and really feel it when you say it.

Next, after you have done your morning hygiene, squeeze a half lemon into a glass of drinking water, about 4 ounces or more. *Wait about 10 minutes before drinking the juice you are about to make for <u>breakfast</u>.* For <u>breakfast,</u> make a bowl of berries and mix with some vegan yogurt made from coconut.

In your juicer, juice 4 stems of celery. *After drinking your juice again, wait at least an hour before eating anything else.* For snacks, have a cup of berries ready.

Read ahead, so you know what you will need for day two.

Do three simple exercises, then write down the

number of reps you did for each one on the next page.

NOTES

_____

_____

_____

_____

_____

_____

_____

_____

_____

_____

_____

_____

_____

_____

_____

_____

_____

_____

_____

_____

_____

_____

_____

_____

After all the information I gathered about the mistreatment of animals, I couldn't continue to eat meat. The more I was aware of, the harder and harder it was to do...

Liam Hemsworth

WEEK TWO - DAY TWO

Step one: start your affirmation, look in the mirror and say <u>thank you for my healthy body,</u> then end it with <u>thank you, thank you, thank you,</u> and really feel it when you say it.

Next, after you have done your morning hygiene, squeeze a half lemon into a glass of drinking water, about 4 ounces or more. *Wait about 10 minutes before drinking the fresh juice you are about to make for <u>breakfast</u>.*

In your juicer, again preferably a masticating juicer, juice 4 stems of celery. *After drinking your juice, wait at least an hour before eating anything else*; a bowl of fruit would be ideal. Each day we will be adding a new ingredient to the juice, so make sure you have got all the ingredients listed above or read ahead, so you know what you will need for the next day. For snacks, eat a cup of berries (any kind will do).

Do three simple exercises, then write down the number of reps you did for each one on the next page.

NOTES

_____
_____
_____
_____
_____
_____
_____
_____
_____
_____
_____
_____
_____
_____
_____
_____
_____
_____
_____
_____
_____
_____
_____
_____

My own view is that being a vegetarian or vegan is not an end in itself, but a means towards reducing both human and animal suffering, and leaving a habitable planet to future generations...

Peter Singer

WEEK TWO - DAY THREE

Step one: start your affirmation, look in the mirror and say <u>thank you for my healthy body,</u> then end it with <u>thank you, thank you, thank you.</u>

Next, after you have done your morning hygiene, squeeze a half lemon into a glass of drinking water, about 4 ounces or more. Use the other half of the lemon for your juice. *Wait for about 10 minutes before drinking the fresh juice you are about to make for <u>breakfast</u>.*

In your juicer, juice 4 stems of celery, half of the lemon, and 1 green apple. After drinking your juice again, wait at least an hour before eating anything else. For snacks, have a cup of grapes. Read ahead, so you know what you will need for tomorrow. As the week goes on, we will be adding to your juice and lunch and eventually dinner.

Do three simple exercises, then write down the number of reps you did for each one on the next page.

NOTES

A vegetarian is a person who won't eat any-thing that can have children...

David Brenner

WEEK TWO - DAY FOUR

Step one: start your affirmation, look in the mirror and say <u>thank you for my healthy body,</u> then end it with <u>thank you, thank you, thank you.</u>

Next, after you have done your morning hygiene, squeeze a half lemon into a glass of drinking water, about 4 ounces or more. *Wait about 10 minutes before drinking the fresh juice you are about to make for <u>breakfast.</u>*

In your juicer, juice 2 stems of celery, half a lemon, 1 green apple, and a half cup of spinach. After drinking your juice again, wait at least an hour before eating anything else. For snacks, have a cup of grapes. Read ahead, so you know what you will need for tomorrow.

Do three simple exercises, then write down the number of reps you did for each one on the next page.

NOTES

Meat is a wasteful use of water and creates a lot of greenhouse gases. It puts enormous pressure on the world's resources. A vegetarian diet is better...

Nicholas Stern

WEEK TWO - DAY FIVE

Step one: start your affirmation, look in the mirror and say <u>thank you for my healthy body,</u> then end it with <u>thank you, thank you, thank you.</u>

Next, after you have done your morning hygiene, squeeze a half lemon into a glass of drinking water, about 4 ounces or more. *Wait about 10 minutes before drinking the fresh juice you are about to make for <u>breakfast</u>.*

In your juicer, juice 2 stems of celery, half a lemon, 1 green apple, half a cup of spinach, and a half cucumber. Refrigerate the other half of the cucumber for tomorrow's juice. After drinking your juice again, wait at least an hour before eating anything else. For snacks, have a cup of berries. Read ahead, so you know what you will need for tomorrow.

Do three simple exercises, then write down the number of reps you did for each one on the next page.

NOTES

Most people see a documentary about the meat industry and then they become a vegetarian for a week...

Jason Reitman

WEEK TWO
- DAY SIX

Step one: start your affirmation, look in the mirror and say <u>thank you for my healthy body,</u> then end it with <u>thank you, thank you, thank you.</u>

Next, after you have done your morning hygiene, squeeze a half lemon into a glass of drinking water, about 4 ounces or more. *Wait about 10 minutes before drinking the fresh juice you are about to make for <u>breakfast.</u>*

In your juicer, juice 2 stems of celery, half a lemon, 1 green apple, half a cup of spinach, and a half cucumber. *After drinking your juice again, wait at least an hour before eating anything else.* For snacks, have a cup of berries.

Side notes; if you are at work during lunchtime, and then prepare your lunch the night before.

For <u>lunch,</u> we will be making quinoa. Follow the direction in the back of the package and season to your liking. To compliment your meal, make a delicious salad that has different leafy greens, half an avocado sliced into cubes, 2 tablespoons of your preferred seeds (pumpkin, flaxseeds, chia seeds, or sunflower) a half of cucumbers thinly sliced, and add about ¼ cup of your favorite oil, ½ a teaspoon of sea salt to taste, mine is extra virgin olive oil with Himalayan salt. You can get creative with your salads. Add tomatoes or some raisins.

About an hour after eating, have either a glass of water or a cup of your favorite tea, sweetened with raw honey. For dessert, have some melon or berries. Read ahead, so you know what you will need for tomorrow.

Do three simple exercises, then write down the number of reps you did for each one on the next page.

NOTES

Being a vegetarian really saves lives...

Esha Gupta

WEEK TWO - DAY SEVEN

Step one: start your affirmation, look in the mirror and say <u>thank you for my healthy body,</u> then end it with <u>thank you, thank you, thank you.</u>

Next, after you have done your morning hygiene, squeeze a half lemon into a glass of drinking water, about 4 ounces or more. *Wait about 10 minutes before drinking the juice you are about to make for <u>breakfast</u>.*

In your juicer, juice 2 stems of celery, half a lemon, 1 green apple, a half cup of spinach, a half cucumber, and a quarter-size piece of ginger root. *After drinking your juice again, wait at least an hour before eating anything else.* For snacks, have a cup of berries ready.

For <u>lunch,</u> pour 1/8 cup of avocado oil in a pan, cook the sliced half onion for about 10 minutes before adding the cabbage and zucchini. Next, cut about ¼ of the green cabbage into slices, slice up one zucchini, and add both ingredients to the pan with the cooked onions. Cook for another 10 minutes. Once done, add to the delicious salad with different leafy greens, half an avocado sliced into cubes, seeds (pumpkin, flaxseeds, chia seeds, or sunflower), cucumbers, and add your favorite oil with sea salt to taste. Finally, add tomatoes or some raisins, or even some types of nuts.

About an hour after eating, either drink a glass of water or a cup of your favorite tea, sweetened with raw honey. For dessert, have some melon or berries.

For <u>dinner,</u> we have spaghetti squash which is high in antioxidants and many other valuable nutrients that I have shared at the beginning of this week. To make spaghetti squash, you will need a somewhat deep baking glass. Add a cup of water to the baking dish. Cut spaghetti squash lengthwise, scoop out the seeds, and bake the squash halves shell-side up in the oven. Be careful cutting your squash; these are hard, dense, sometimes slippery little guys—and they're tough to slice through. While your squash is baking, cook some fresh-cut carrots and beets, add 2 tablespoons olive oil, sprinkled garlic salt, and a cup of water, cover until well done. In a cooking pan, you will add one small can of tomato paste; 1/4 cup of extra virgin olive oil, 4 basil leaves, one sliced tomato, and one can of tomato sauce. Finally, add about a teaspoon of garlic salt. Mix well and cook for about 10 minutes, stirring frequently. Check on your carrots and beets and stir as needed. They should be done by the time your squash is ready. Once Spaghetti squash is done, take a fork, and you will scrape out the meat of the squash. It will come off like noodles hence the name. Place the amount you will be eating onto your plate and top it off with the sauce you just made. Now your plate is ready for your added beets and carrots.

Make a salad on the side again using olive oil and salt to taste. About an hour after eating, have either a glass of water or a cup of your favorite tea, sweetened with raw honey.

Congratulations, you have now finished your second week, on to the next.

Read ahead, so you know what you will need for tomorrow.

Do three simple exercises, then write down the number of reps you did for each one on the next page.

NOTES

INGREDIENTS FOR THE THIRD WEEK

We have now reached our last week. Whew! That was easy. You can repeat the process and even mix and match the recipes to your liking.

BENEFITS

Lemons contain high levels of vitamin C and are quite effective in curing digestion problems. They also carry digestive juices that relieve you from things like heartburn, bloating, belching, and gastric problems. By taking lemon with fresh warm water in the morning, it aids in proper digestion. It removes toxins from the kidneys and the digestive system. It is good for high blood pressure, Cold and fevers, respiratory disorders, dental health, weight loss, and so much more.

Oranges contain vitamin C, fiber, potassium, choline, which are all good for your heart! Potassium, an electrolyte mineral, is vital for allowing electricity to flow through your body, which helps keep your heart beating.

Turmeric root has been used for medicinal purposes for nearly 4,000 years. It reduces inflammation. It helps with pain management and is great for the skin. Turmeric is also rich in vitamin C, B6, and other antioxidants that reduce heart disease and diabetes risk. In addition, it is an excellent source of Manganese, Iron, Potassium, Omega-3 fatty acids, and fiber.

Ginger boosts your immune system, relieves nausea, and has a healing effect on your digestive system. Ginger reduces blood pressure, and Cholesterol and stimulates the heart. Ginger is more powerful than onions or garlic. It's known to fight inflammation and viruses and destroys the cancer stem cell. It is also known to lower cholesterol.

Strawberries are bursting with vitamins, minerals and great when fighting cancer. They are rich in vitamin C and other antioxidants, Potassium, Magnesium, Calcium, vitamin K, and fiber.

Bananas are a great source of vitamin B, Magnesium, potassium, also rich in probiotics.

Blueberries have an impressive ray of antioxidants, enhance vitamin C, and are great when fighting cancer.

Raw Honey is antibacterial and antifungal, packed with antioxidants, and can lower blood pressure. Raw honey contains sodium and potassium, calcium and magnesium, phosphorus and selenium, copper, zinc, iron, manganese and chromium, B vitamins, Vitamin C and K. You get the picture. It's good for you, but not for children under 1 year of age.

Yams are associated with many other health benefits, including; improved digestive health. Studies indicate that the resistant starch in yams may increase digestive enzymes that help break down food and increase good bacteria. As a result, they can be particularly helpful in fighting a battle with breast cancer. In addition, because sweet potatoes and yams contain vitamins A, B6, C, and E, they are a healthy choice for disease prevention.

Onions are high in vitamin C that's involved in regulating immune health, collagen production, tissue repair, and the absorption of iron.

Olive oil helps clear the blood of toxins, balances your cholesterol. It's anti-inflammatory, antibacterial, heart-healthy, and skin-healthy.

Wild rice improves digestion and heart health, stimulates growth and repair throughout the body, slows the signs of aging, protects against chronic diseases, prevents the onset of diabetes, strengthens bones, and boosts the immune system. It's rich in antioxidants and gluten-free. In addition, it contains potassium, phosphorus, zinc, magnesium, and folate, which are in the vitamin B family.

Sea salt, not all salt is created equal, and there is a difference between unrefined, mineral-rich varieties like sea salt versus salt that has been heavily processed and stripped of its natural nutrients. Sea salts are a great source of micronutrients. Sea salt contains many of the major electrolytes, like sodium, magnesium, calcium, and potassium, essential to good health. Regular table salt is stripped from those essential nutrients.

Leafy greens support brain function, make your skin glow, relieve stress, support bone health, boost digestive enzymes, and support your immune system. You can find many studies on the health benefits of eating leafy greens. You have a variety to pick from. I personally love mixing several. Here are a few to list, kale, spinach, arugula, and chard, to name a few.

Avocado is incredibly nutritious. Some of the nutrients; vitamin K, Folate, vitamin C, Potassium, vitamin B5, vitamin B6, and vitamin E, to name a few. Avocados are loaded with fiber. Eating avocados can lower your cholesterol and triglyceride levels and may even relieve symptoms of arthritis.

Cucumber, carry protein, fiber, vitamin C, vitamin K, magnesium, and potassium. Cucumbers also contain antioxidants that block oxidation. It promotes hydration and may aid in weight loss and lower blood sugar.

Portobello mushrooms can help reduce estrogen levels in the body, thus preventing breast cancer, antidiabetic. Portobello mushroom is nutrient-rich therefore it has various types of vitamins like A, D, B complex, and high dietary fibers. They help in the prevention of heart-related diseases. This mushroom contains a compound called lovastatin. Portobello mushrooms are antibacterial and antifungal. They have antioxidant properties. Rich source of protein and Improves memory.

Watermelon's health benefits are vast and include preventing diseases and disorders, including kidney disorders, high blood pressure, cancer, diabetes, heart diseases, heat stroke, macular degeneration, and even impotence. The watermelon seeds that you would chew up and eat are low in calories and high in nutrients, and no, they are not poisonous though they may be hard to digest for some. Instead, they boost heart health and immunity and keep your blood sugar levels under control. In addition, the seeds are rich in numerous micronutrients like potassium, copper, selenium, and zinc – nutrients that you may not obtain from your diet in adequate quantities.

Eating the seeds directly from the fruit is good, but the sprouted ones are better. Just about 1/8 cup of the seeds offer about 10 grams of protein. Sprouting the seeds also removes the compounds in the seeds that make them harder to be absorbed by the body. So if you prefer to sprout them, instead go for it but don't throw them away. I eat them fresh from the melon but sprouting them is also very beneficial.

Celery is great in hydration; it also contains vitamins A, K, C, E, and B vitamins. It carries compounds that may help with inflammation in the body, help in lowering cholesterol levels and reduce blood pressure. Boost your immune system and reduce pain. The list is way too long, but you get the picture.

Green apple promotes weight loss, improves hair quality, great on skin health, protects our vision, and improves digestion. Digestion is the answer to our overall health, as it is through our digestion, we receive our nutrition. If we have joint problems, green apples have been known to strengthen our joints. Green apples are also known to detoxify the liver. This is important since the liver does over five hundred functions for the body. Now we can see why the old saying goes *An Apple a Day Keeps the Doctor Away.* I mean, when you look up information on the health benefits of green apples, we also learn it can prevent asthma, strengthens the immune system, and on and on it goes.

Spinach is great for the eyes, relieving high blood pressure, gout, arthritis, heart diseases and helping in the proper functioning of the brain. It carries antioxidants, vitamin C, Anthocyanin, and Folate, as well as Quercetin. Aids in digestion and are beneficial for our skin and eyes.

Veganism is not a "sacrifice." It is a joy...

Gary L. Francione

WEEK THREE
– DAY ONE

As we come to our last week, continue to affirm your health daily as you have for the last three weeks. Make sure to look in the mirror and then thank yourself for all that you do.

Step one: start your affirmation, look in the mirror and say <u>thank you for my healthy body,</u> then end it with <u>thank you, thank you, thank you,</u> and really feel it when you say it.

Next, after you have done your morning hygiene, squeeze a half lemon into a glass of drinking water, about 4 ounces or more. *Then wait 10 minutes before drinking the juice you are about to make for <u>breakfast</u>.*

In your juicer, juice 2 oranges, and half a lemon. *After drinking your juice again, wait at least an hour before eating anything else.* For snacks, have a cup of berries ready. If you want to have a piece of toast, make sure it is all grain bread.

Read ahead so you know what you will need for day two.

Do three simple exercises, then write down the number of reps you did for each one on the next page.

NOTES

If slaughterhouses had glass walls, the whole world would be vegetarian...

Linda McCartney

WEEK THREE
– DAY TWO

Step one: start your affirmation, look in the mirror and say <u>thank you for my healthy body,</u> then complete it with <u>thank you, thank you, thank you,</u> and really feel it when you say it.

Next, after you have done your morning hygiene, squeeze a half lemon into a glass of drinking water, about 4 ounces or more. *Wait about 10 minutes before drinking the fresh juice you are about to make for <u>breakfast</u>.*

In your juicer, preferably a masticating juicer, juice 2 oranges, half a lemon, 1 turmeric root. *After drinking the juice, wait at least an hour before eating anything else.* Each day we will be adding a new ingredient to the juice, so make sure you have gotten all the ingredients listed above or read ahead, so you know what you will need for the next day. For snacks, eat a cup of berries (any kind will do).

Do three simple exercises, then write down the number of reps you did for each one on the next page.

NOTES

I like animals, all animals. I wouldn't hurt a cat or a dog – or a chicken or a cow. And I wouldn't ask someone else to hurt them for me. That's why I'm a vegetarian...

Peter Dinklage

WEEK THREE – DAY THREE

Step one: start your affirmation, look in the mirror and say <u>thank you for my healthy body,</u> then end it with <u>thank you, thank you, thank you.</u>

Next, after you have done your morning hygiene, squeeze a half lemon into a glass of drinking water, about 4 ounces or more. Use the other half of the lemon for your juice. *Wait about for 10 minutes before drinking the fresh juice you are about to make for* <u>*breakfast.*</u>

In your juicer, juice 2 oranges, half a lemon, 1 turmeric root, and a small piece of ginger root about the size of a quarter. After drinking your juice again, wait at least an hour before eating anything else. For snacks, have a cup of berries ready.

Do three simple exercises, then write down the number of reps you did for each one on the next page.

NOTES

If you don't like seeing pictures of violence towards animals being posted, you need to help stop the violence, not the pictures...

Johnny Depp

WEEK THREE – DAY FOUR

Step one: start your affirmation, look in the mirror and say <u>thank you for my healthy body,</u> then end it with <u>thank you, thank you, thank you.</u>

Next, after you have done your morning hygiene, squeeze a half lemon into a glass of drinking water, about 4 ounces or more. *Wait about 10 minutes before drinking the fresh juice you are about to make for <u>breakfast</u>.*

In your juicer, juice 2 oranges, half a lemon, 1 turmeric root, and a small piece of ginger root. *After drinking your juice again, wait at least an hour before eating a cup of seeded watermelon.* For snacks, have a banana ready. Read ahead, so you know what you will need for tomorrow.

Do three simple exercises, then write down the number of reps you did for each one on the next page.

NOTES

_____

_____

_____

_____

_____

_____

_____

_____

_____

_____

_____

_____

_____

_____

_____

_____

_____

_____

_____

_____

_____

_____

The love for all living creatures is the most noble attribute of man...

Charles Darwin

WEEK THREE – DAY FIVE

Step one: start your affirmation, look in the mirror and say <u>thank you for my healthy body,</u> then end it with <u>thank you, thank you, thank you.</u>

Next, after you have done your morning hygiene, squeeze a half lemon into a glass of drinking water, about 4 ounces or more. *Wait about 10 minutes before drinking the fresh juice you are about to make for <u>breakfast</u>.*

In your juicer, juice 2 stems of celery, half a lemon, 1 green apple, half a cup of spinach, and a half cucumber. Refrigerate the other half of the cucumber for tomorrow's juice. *After drinking your juice again, wait at least an hour before eating anything else.* For snacks, have a cup of berries ready. Read ahead, so you know what you will need for tomorrow.

Do three simple exercises, then write down the number of reps you did for each one on the next page.

NOTES

We can judge the heart of a man by his treatment of animals...

Immanuel Kant

WEEK THREE
– DAY SIX

Step one: start your affirmation, look in the mirror and say <u>thank you for my healthy body,</u> then end it with <u>thank you, thank you, thank you.</u>

Next, after you have done your morning hygiene, squeeze a half lemon into a glass of drinking water, about 4 ounces or more. Wait about 10 minutes before drinking the fresh juice you are about to make for <u>breakfast.</u>

In your juicer, juice 2 stems of celery, half a lemon, 1 green apple, half a cup of spinach, and a half cucumber. After drinking your juice again, wait at least an hour before eating anything else. For snacks, have a cup of berries ready.

Side notes; if you are at work during lunch-time, and then prepare your lunch the night before.

For <u>lunch,</u> make a delicious salad that has different leafy greens, half an avocado sliced into cubes, 2 tablespoons of your preferred seeds (pumpkin, flaxseeds, chia seeds, or sunflower) a half of cucumbers thinly sliced, and add about ¼ cup of your favorite oil, ½ teaspoon of sea salt to taste; mine is extra virgin olive oil with Himalayan salt. You can get creative with your salads. Add tomatoes or some raisins.

About an hour after eating, drink either a glass of water or a cup of your favorite tea, sweetened with raw honey. For dessert, have some melon or berries. Read ahead, so you know what you will need for tomorrow.

Do three simple exercises, then write down the number of reps you did for each one on the next page.

NOTES

I did not become a vegetarian for my health; I did it for the health of the chickens...

Isaac Bashevis Singer

WEEK THREE –
DAY SEVEN

Step one: start your affirmation, look in the mirror and say <u>thank you for my healthy body,</u> then end it with <u>thank you, thank you, thank you.</u>

Next, after you have done your morning hygiene, squeeze a half lemon into a glass of drinking water, about 4 ounces or more. *After drinking your lemon water, wait 10 minutes before drinking the juice you are about to make for <u>breakfast</u>.*

In your juicer, juice 2 stems of celery, half a lemon, one green apple, a half cup of spinach, a half cucumber, and about a quarter-size piece of ginger root. *After drinking your juice again, wait at least an hour before eating anything else.* For snacks, have a cup of berries ready.

For <u>lunch,</u> add some mixed cooked vegetables to your salad that has different leafy greens, a half an avocado sliced into cubes, seeds (pumpkin, flaxseeds, chia seeds, or sunflower) cucumbers, and add your favorite oil with sea salt to taste. Add tomatoes or some raisins or even some types of nuts.

About an hour after eating, drink either a glass

of water or a cup of your favorite tea, sweetened with raw honey. For dessert, have some melon or berries.

For <u>dinner,</u> we are having yams, onions, wild rice, and Portobello mushrooms.

Peel your yams, cut into medium slices and boil in water until tender. Slice onion and place in a pan with olive oil and cook until translucent. Take the Portobello mushrooms with some olive oil, sprinkled with sea salt, and place in a covered baking dish and cook for about 30 minutes or until well done. Now cook your wild rice following instructions on the back of the package; add about 1 teaspoon of sea salt for every cup of rice. Rice is usually ready in 15 minutes. Mix the cooked yams and onions with its oil and sprinkle some sea salt. And now you are ready to serve yourself.

For dessert, put together sliced strawberries and banana, blueberries, and lightly dress it with raw honey. About an hour after eating, have either a glass of water or a cup of your favorite tea, sweetened with raw honey.

Eating clean is essential to good health and that is what these steps were about. Congratulations, you have now finished your three-week step into a healthier you.

Now do your three simple exercises, then write down the number of reps you did for each one on the next page.

Cheers to good health!

NOTES

_____
_____
_____
_____
_____
_____
_____
_____
_____
_____
_____
_____
_____
_____
_____
_____
_____
_____
_____
_____
_____

BOOKS BY THIS AUTHOR

Our Journey To Option C: An Inspirational Love Story That Proves That Love Does Conquer All...Including Cancer

Cancer doesn't have to be a death sentence. In this book Our Journey To Option C you will find the story of a very courageous couple and their struggle to fight her cancer with whatever worked best for her. It is an excellent read. You will encounter almost certain death, a desperate fight to survive and an indomitable spirit and will to win the battle. You will be encouraged to seek what is best for you in whatever your battlefield is, because Option C is not limited to only cancer or even only to disease. It is a guiding principal for any struggle or problem life may throw at you. You will be blessed by the courageous story that is written within these pages. Dr. Dan Rogers, M.D., Ph.D., N.M.D., FMCM Founder of the GersonPlus Therapy and Rogers

Therapy.Lourdes Colón was a single mother and a successful actress when she met Chris LaVoy. He was the stage director for the theatrical production that she was a part of and the two fell in love. Just as Lourdes was set to explode into Hollywood her world was turned upside down when she was diagnosed with cancer. Their world was torn apart at the diagnosis, but their marriage was tested when Lourdes revealed to her husband that she was going to fight her cancer naturally, and that she was going to document her healing so that the world could see that there was a way to beat cancer without poison or harmful side effects. Lourdes learned about the human body and cancer. Through trial and error Lourdes learned how she could get whole. Lourdes faced resistance from friends and family, but still had that strength to move forward on a journey that took her all the way to Mexico, and to death's door, where she was greeted with messages from the other side from "Light Beings".Our Journey to Option C is a book that surpasses a cancer survivor's story and transcends to life lessons and a mindset that allows for Lourdes and Chris to live their lives richer and with more meaning than ever before.

NOTES

NOTES

NOTES

Made in the USA
Las Vegas, NV
05 March 2022